Home Remedies

For

Dengue And Malaria

Home Remedies

For

Dengue And Malaria

By Monica Sidoine,
S.N.H.S. Dip. Herbalism

DISCLAIMER

This book is to serve as an informational guide for use in the home. The remedies and procedures contained in this book are meant to supplement and are not intended to be a substitute for professional medical care. Please seek a qualified medical practitioner for all ailments. The author nor distributors takes no responsibility for customers choosing to treat themselves. Your use of this information is at your own risk.

ISBN - 13: 978-1534986718
ISBN - 10: 1534986715

Proof Read by Jasmine Ned Anunda

Printed By Create Space Publishing
United States of America

ACKNOWLEDGMENTS

I would like to thank all those who have contributed in one way or another to the completion of HOME REMEDIES FOR DENGUE AND MALARIA.

I thank God for giving me the vision, wisdom and good health to write this book. For all he has done and will continue to do in my life.

For the many prayer warriors who interceded on behalf of this project and also their moral support.

I thank my daughter Jasmine Ned Anunda for proof reading.

Thank you all.

Monica Sidoine.

PREFACE

The procedures in this Book was designed to be as simple as possible so that anyone will be able to follow them. Most of the items used are local things which you would either have at home, in your kitchen garden or can be easily purchased from the local market or health store for a very low cost.

By using the simple remedies and health tips outlined in this book it should help you in your journey to recovery from Dengue and Malaria.

TABLE OF CONTENTS

DENGUE

Dengue is a tropical disease caused by a virus that is transmitted by the Aedes aegypti mosquitoes.

It is found in rural and suburban areas.

The symptoms are:
High fever.
Mild skin rash.
Slow pulse.
Facial congestion.
A decrease in the blood pressure.
Severe muscle and joint pains.
Abdominal and lower back pains.
Headaches and soreness in the eye balls.
Mild nausea and excessive vomiting.
Bleeding from the nostrils.

The symptoms occur between 3 – 10 days after been bitten by the Aedes aegypti mosquito. It can last up to 10 days. Recovery would usually take several weeks.

NATURAL REMEDIES

- Take 1 teaspoon of lemon juice three times daily.

- Remove the stalks from 2 large fresh papaya leaves, pound to squeeze the juice from the leaves. It should yield about 2 tablespoons of juice.
  Drink it once daily.

- Drink ½ cup of apple juice three times daily.

- Steep 1oz of ginger in 1 liter of boiling water for 20 minutes. Drink 1 cup three times daily.

- Steep 10 neem leaves in 1 liter of boiling water for 30 minutes.
  Drink 1 cup four times daily.

- Steep 1oz of barley grass in 1 liter of boiling water for 30 minutes.
  Drink 1 cup 3 times daily.

- Steep 1 yellow papaya leaf in 3 cups of boiling water for 30 minutes.
  Drink 1 cup three times daily.

- Steep 5 basil leaves in 2 cups of boiling water for 20 minutes. Drink 1 cup twice daily.

- Steep 1oz of fenugreek in 1 liter of boiling water for 30 minutes.
  Drink 1 cup 4 times daily.

- Steep 1oz of goldenseal in 1 liter of boiling water for 30 minutes.
  Drink 1 cup three times daily.

- Steep 1oz of coriander in 1 liter of boiling water for 30 minutes.
  Drink 1 cup 4 times daily.

- Drink 1 glass of orange juice twice daily.

- Drink 1 glass of pomegranate juice twice daily.

- Drink at least 8 – 10 glasses of water daily.

- Chew same basil leaves daily.

- Chew some barley grass daily.

- Put an icebag on the head to help ease the headache.

- Apply hot Fomentations to the areas where there is pain.

- Apply a Cold Mitten Friction daily after the acute symptoms have gone.
  See the Hydrotherapy section for Fomentations and Cold Mitten Friction.

- When the fever is high, have tepid sponges.

- Have enemas.

Health Tips

- Eat lots of raw garlic and onions at least three times daily.

- Chew ginger root at least three times daily.

- Use oregano in your cooking.

- Have a light diet.

- Take lots of rest in bed to help with the recovery.

- Use a mosquito repellant especially when going out.

- Use a mosquito net when going to bed.

- Make sure that your hands and legs are covered.

- Avoid dark coloured clothing which will attract mosquitos.

- Get rid of any water which is lying around the home.

MALARIA

Malaria is an infectious disease caused by Plasmodium which is a parasite that is transmitted by the bite of infected female Anopheles mosquitoes. It is found in tropical countries.

There are four types – P. falciparum, P. vivax, P. malariae, and P. ovale.

P. vivax, P. malariae and P. ovale can remain in the liver for years in a dormant state with no symptoms. If the immune system drops it can reenter the blood stream anytime, even after dozens of years. When this happens it can cause another active case of malaria to develop.

P. falciparum is the most deadly form of malaria, it causes a high fever and it does not relapse longer than 6 months. The two deadly complications of it are Cerebral Malaria and Blackwater Fever.

Cerebral Malaria can cause an obstruction of blood flow to the brain which can result to a lack of oxygen there. It can cause mental confusion, coma and death.

In Blackwater Fever blood is passed out through the urine causing it to be red or black and the skin can have a yellow colour. It can cause kidney failure and death after, if it is not treated urgently.

Some symptoms of Malaria are:
Recurring chills for several hours, fever every 1 – 3 days.
Sleepiness, enemia, weakness, nausea and vomiting.
Headaches, perspiring profusely, sensitivity to light.
Abdominal pain and diarrhea; lack of appetite and sore throat.
Backaches and muscle pains; joint and bone pain.
The symptoms can occur about 10 days after the bite.

NATURAL REMEDIES

- Boil 1oz of star anise in 1 liter of boiling water for 30 minutes.
  Drink 1 cup three times daily.

- Steep 5 basil leaves in 2 cups of boiling water for 20 minutes.
  Drink 1 cup twice daily.

- Boil 1oz ginger root in 1liter of water for 15 minutes.
  Drink 1 cup three times daily.

- Steep 1oz of cinnamon in 1 liter of boiling water for 15 minutes.
  Drink I cup 4 times daily.

- Steep 1oz of cinchona tree bark in 1 liter of boiling water for 1 hour.
  Drink 1 cup 4 times daily before meals.

- Steep 2 teaspoons of powdered cinchona tree bark in 1 liter of boiling water for 30 minutes.
  Drink 1 cup 4 times daily before meals.

- Steep 10 neem leaves in 1 liter of boiling water for 30 minutes.
  Drink 1 cup four times daily.

- Stir 1 tablespoon of charcoal in a glass of water.
  Drink 1 glass three times daily.

- Steep 1 yellow papaya leaf in 3 cups of boiling water for 30 minutes.
  Drink 1 cup three times daily.

- Steep 1oz of goldenseal in 1 liter of boiling water for 30 minutes.
  Drink 1 cup 3 times daily.

- Steep 1oz of Echinacea in 1 liter of boiling water for 30 minutes.
  Drink 1 cup 4 times daily.

- Drink about 12 glasses of water daily.

- Drink lots of orange juice throughout the day.

- Cut 1 grapefruit with the skin into pieces. Boil it in 1 liter of water for 10 minutes.
  Drink 1 cup 3 times daily.

- Drink the juice of one lemon with some water on the morning of the first day. Build up the dosage of lemons by one lemon daily until nine lemons are taken with water for the day. Decrease the dosage by one lemon per day until the entire treatment period of 18 days is completed.

- Eat 12 papaya seeds three times daily. They can be eaten fresh or dried. The fresh seeds can be placed outdoors in the sun to air dry or put in the oven for a few minutes, cool and store in a zip lock bag.

- Eat 1 large steamed onion daily.

- Eat 1 whole steamed garlic bulb daily.

- When the first symptoms appear eat 5 raw garlic cloves 3 times daily.

- Eat lots of grapefruits daily.

- Go on a vegetarian diet.

- Eat fresh pineapple every day if possible.

- Eat walnuts, flaxseeds and any other nuts or seeds.

- Take a warm water enema.

- Apply a warm Fomentation to the low chest and abdomen ½ hour to 2 hours before the fever comes on. In between the fomentations do a Cold Mitten Friction to the body starting with the upper extremities down to the lower extremities. Turnover and end with the cold mitten friction to the back. Rest for at least one hour.

- Apply a Cold Mitten Friction every two hours, with hot and cold to the spine, to tone up the nervous system.
  See the Hydrotherapy Formulas Section for Cold Mitten Friction and Fomentation.

- **During the fever:** Apply Cold applications – sponges.

- **During the chills:** Apply Hot applications – hot packs.

Health Tips

- Exercise twice daily for at least 30 minutes or until you sweat.

- Get at least 7 hours of sleep nightly.

- Get lots of fresh air daily.

- Have a healthy diet.

- Abstain from all dairy products

- Decrease on the intake of sugar, fats and chocolate.

- Use a mosquito repellant especially when going out.

- Use a mosquito net when going to bed.

- Make sure that your hands and legs are covered.

- Avoid dark coloured clothing which will attract mosquitos.

- Get rid of any water which is lying around the home.

- Still continue with the treatments three days after the symptoms have gone.

HYDROTHERAPY TREATMENTS

FOMENTATIONS

HERBAL TEA FOMENTATION:

1. Make an infusion or decoction.

2. Dip a towel folded in 2 or 3 layers the size of the body area you want to cover in the solution.

3. Wring out the excess liquid. Apply it to the affected area of the body.

4. Place a thick towel over the fomentation to help retain the heat longer.

5. Keep the tea hot and change the cloths every 3 minutes. Do 5 rounds.

6. End with a cold towel rub to the area.

Cold Mitten Friction

It increases heat production, restores tone to blood vessels and muscles, helps with the elimination of toxins.

Items needed:

Two or more towels.

Friction mitts: You can use a washcloth wrapped around the hand or make mitts by sewing a folded washcloth along the side and the top.

Bucket of very cold water.

Procedure:

1. Begin with the right hand. Dip the mitten or washcloth in cold water and squeeze out the excess.

2. Rub the part vigorously until a red glow develops, avoiding skin lesions or painful areas.

3. Dry thoroughly and cover.

4. Move to another part and repeat the procedure taking one part after another until the entire body surface has been covered.

Other Book Titles by the Same Author

Can be viewed at this link:
http://www.amazon.com/author/monicasidoine

Healing Poultices

The Top 20 Most Valuable Herbs

Home Remedies For Cancer

Home Remedies For Losing Weight

Home Remedies For Blood Pressure and Diabetes

Home Remedies For Headaches and Insomnia

Home Remedies For Sinusitis and Tonsillitis

Home Remedies For Constipation and Diarrhea

Home Remedies For Asthma and Bronchitis

Home Remedies For Dehydration and Vomiting

Home Remedies For Pneumonia and Tuberculosis

Home Remedies For Stress, Depression and Anxiety

NOTES

NOTES

NOTES

www.ingramcontent.com/pod-product-compliance
Lightning Source LLC
Chambersburg PA
CBHW061953280526
45787CB00004B/1849